MW01195713

Candlemaking Aromatherapy: The Ultimate Guide to Combining Candle Making and Aromatherapy to Beat Stress, Promote Weight Loss, and Heal Common Problems

All rights Reserved. No part of this publication or the information in it may be quoted from or reproduced in any form by means such as printing, scanning, photocopying or otherwise without prior written permission of the copyright holder.

Disclaimer and Terms of Use: Effort has been made to ensure that the information in this book is accurate and complete, however, the author and the publisher do not warrant the accuracy of the information, text and graphics contained within the book due to the rapidly changing nature of science, research, known and unknown facts and internet. The Author and the publisher do not hold any responsibility for errors, omissions or contrary interpretation of the subject matter herein. This book is presented solely for motivational and informational purposes only.

Summary

Candle making is something that has been practiced for many years for different reasons. One of those reasons is aromatherapy. It is now possible to use candles to help you lose weight, relieve stress and so on. This is a practice that has fast gained popularity due to the fact that more people are leaning towards natural remedies for their illnesses and discomforts.

People have being buying these aromatherapy candles but the good news is that you can now make your own and we will show you how to go about it using the different recipes. We'll look at the facts you need to know before you even start the process of making aromatherapy candles. We will give you important information on the fragrances for aromatherapy candle making and the merits and demerits of making your own aromatherapy candles as opposed to buying. We'll get in to the instructions you should follow to ensure that you make good aromatherapy candles and in a safe way. This book is aimed at equipping you with the information you need to use candle aromatherapy for your worries.

Table of Contents

Introduction

Are you aware that candles can be used for aromatherapy? Well, it is possible and more people are realizing the benefits of this. Making aromatherapy candles is a process you will enjoy. It is an activity that is both unique and beneficial. Aromatherapy uses natural aromas and fragrances as the name suggests for ensuring the well-being of your body. It involves the use of essential oils with useful medicinal properties. The essential oils are from flowers, roots, fruits and plants extracts. There is a huge variety of the essential oils reaching up to around a hundred and fifty different types.

When done correctly, aromatherapy can provide both physical and psychological benefits to its users. These different essential oils can be used in various forms such as mouthwashes, soaps and candles. Inhalation, massage and topical application are other ways of practicing aromatherapy too.

Aromatherapy candles are mostly used by people who cannot get time for the topical applications or massage. When you light these candles, they give out the fragrance of the particular essential oil used to manufacture them. This leads to a calm and soothing effect on the environment. When you inhale the aroma then your nasal passage helps your blood stream to absorb the essential oils.

Chapter 1: Merits and demerits of making aromatherapy candles

You may be in the business of making candles for aromatherapy or you might just be in the habit of using them yourself. Either way, you should consider the option of making your own candles as opposed to buying. Making candles can be a great hobby which you can even turn in to a business to earn you some money. It has also been known to be a great way of relieving stress. There are advantages you can enjoy when you make your own candles for aromatherapy.

Save you lots of money

One of the advantages you will enjoy when you decide to make your own candles is the fact that you will end up saving lots of money. You may still buy candles in order to be up to speed with what's new in the market but it won't be expensive because you will be having the candles you need for aromatherapy.

You choose what you want

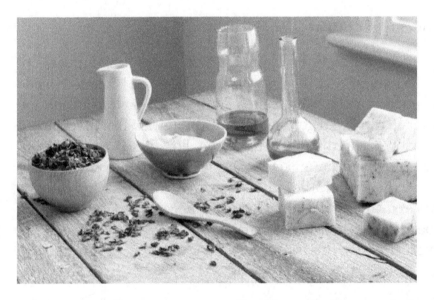

When you make your own candles then you have a choice in the ingredients you use as opposed to when you buy them. When you buy candles, you may get a great type that you like but find that it is missing a particular ingredient that you prefer. You can choose to rectify this by buying the ingredients you want and using them to make your own candles.

As amazing as it is to make your own candles for aromatherapy, there are some disadvantages associated with it too.

It can be messy

Candle making is not one of the neatest hobbies. This is due to the fact that the process of making the candles can turn out to be messy. Although it is quite easy to clean up the mess from the soy waxes, the paraffin can spread to almost every surface. Candle making requires you to work with hot items too. If you are someone who cooks a lot then you may not see this as a big deal but if you don't then it might prove to be a bit cumbersome.

You can get burnt

You may wonder if you should put on gloves in the process of candle making and the answer is no. The wax is melted inside the pouring pots. This melted wax is then poured inside the jars. You can avoid getting burnt if you refrain from picking up the jars when they still have the hot waxes inside them. Therefore, you can make candles without getting burns if you follow the right procedure. However, you just have to be prepared for the fact that you might get burnt at one point especially when you are starting out. When you become an expert at it then this is not something you will worry about.

Chapter 2: What you need to know before you start making aromatherapy candles

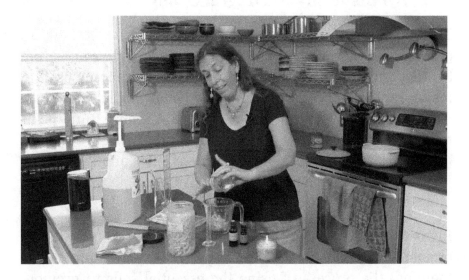

Aromatherapy is thriving as a form of alternative medicine. The aromas contained in the essential oils used for aromatherapy have anti-inflammatory, anti-depressant and pain-relieving properties among others. This is why they are able to alleviate psychological problems such as depression, tension and anxiety. It is necessary for the contents of the essential oils to get in to your blood stream for you to enjoy these benefits. When you apply the essential oils to your skin, it can treat problems such as acne. In addition to that, the oils can also heal burns and wounds. Ensure that the essential oils you use are manufactured using natural raw materials to ensure they are safe and effective.

The most commonly asked question among those interested in aromatherapy candles is how to make them. This is something that is quite possible. However, there is information that you need to have before you start making the aromatherapy candles because it will guide you and ensure that you achieve what you want.

1. Synthetic oils and fragrance oils

The first important thing you should know is how to differentiate essential oils from synthetic fragrance oil. Synthetic fragrance refers to the oil that is commonly used to make candles and is made using man made materials. Essential oils on the other hand originate from natural plant materials. You can use the essential oils to improve your overall health and treat illnesses such as colds and flu even by just inhaling the scents. You can have them in your home, office or even in the car.

In order for you to enjoy the therapeutic benefits of aromatherapy, you have to use essential oils. Aromatherapy is therefore the process of using the essential soils to promote various health benefits. Examples of essential oils commonly used to make these candles include tea tree, Chamomile, lavender, Eucalyptus and peppermint. Citrus oil can be used too because of the amazing smell it gives off.

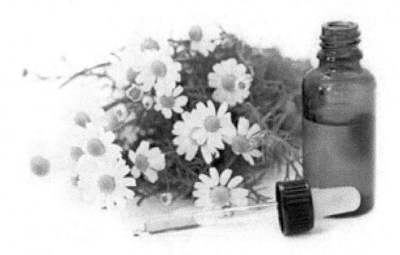

2. Types of essential oils to be used

Before you start making aromatherapy candles you should know that there are essential oils that shouldn't appear as ingredients in the process because they are not safe for use. It is important to know that not everything natural is safe for you. There are some essential oils that may be hazardous to your health.

In addition to that, not every essential oil can be used in candle making. Some essential oils don't have a pleasant smell while others contain components that can irritate the respiratory passages and the mucus membranes.

3. Standard materials required

If you are someone who likes fun and fulfilling hobbies then aromatherapy candle making is for you. If you like making beautiful things then you should try it too. Imagine creating functional personalized candles? It is quite an experience. There are some standard materials needed for you to make aromatherapy candles and examples include a scale, thermometer, candle making molds, goggles, measuring utensils, aprons, pot holders and various safety equipment. There are other materials that vary from one recipe to another.

4. Type of wax recommended

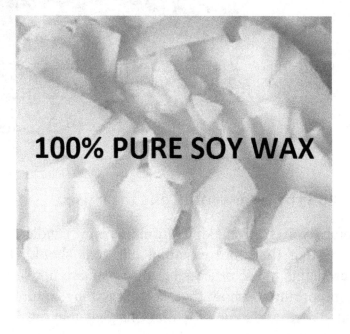

Soy wax is highly recommended among aromatherapy candle makers. This is because it is able to disperse fragrance better. It has a low melting point due to the fact that hydrogenated soybean oil is the ingredient used to make the wax. Therefore it is easier to work with.

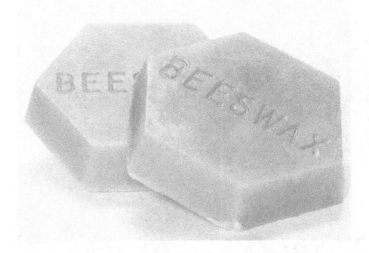

The candles made using soy wax burn more cleanly compared to the ones made using paraffin wax. In addition to that, soy wax burns for longer and is a natural product while paraffin wax is a byproduct of the process of gasoline manufacturing. Soy candles are renewable and quite earth friendly. It is also easy to get the soy wax due to the fact that there are companies producing it in the United States. This doesn't mean that you cannot use the paraffin wax but its best to be aware of the challenges you might face. Beeswax candles are good natural alternatives.

5. Choosing the colors

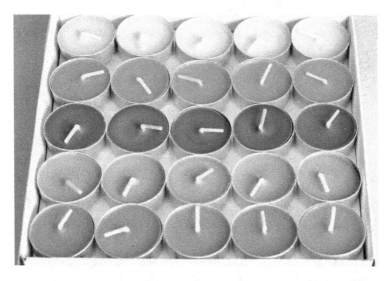

One tip you can apply when choosing colors for the candles is to go for the ones that match with the particular fragrance you are using. For example, you can choose a purple color for an aromatherapy candle made of lavender essential oil and yellow or orange colors for candles made of grapefruit, lemongrass and ginger.

6. Material for the wick

You need to think of the material used to make the wick. Bear in mind that aromatherapy candles should give you health benefits. Therefore good natural fiber wick material is recommended for making the wick. This is why it is advisable to make your purchase from reputable sources.

More craft stores are coming up these days so lots of candle making supplies are quite easy to find.

7. Equipment and supplies

There are various types of soy wax candles you can make depending on what you want. This will also determine the equipment and supplies you will need. Examples of the type of soy candles you can make include tarts for burners, the pillar type candles or container candles. Most people settle for container candles because they are the easiest type to make. You don't have to worry about making a mess because it is easy to clean up soy wax with soap and water. Aromatherapy jar candles are one of the simplest forms of aromatherapy candles to make so you can keep your jelly jars well and all you will have to do is recycle them.

8. Fragrances and dyes

There are specific fragrances and dyes meant for soy wax candles and you can use them if you want. Ensure you choose high quality oils which are strong enough and specifically meant for soy candles. Soy wax is available in either soft blocks or flakes. It is advisable to buy the one in flakes because it will be easy to measure it with regards to the amount you need for various projects. Regardless of whether you are using soy wax, beeswax or paraffin wax, it is important to get the most suitable fragrances and dyes for your candles.

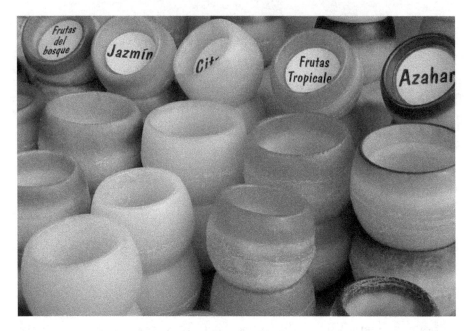

After putting the above facts in to consideration, you can now start the process of making aromatherapy candles.

Chapter 3: Aromatherapy Candle making recipes

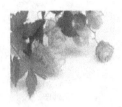

Aromatherapy Recipes

Aromatherapy candles have various uses. They can be used to reduce stress, treat skin problems, give you that calming effect or even help you reduce weight.

There are different recipes you can use to make various aromatherapy candles and they are as follows. It is advisable to have a variety of them at your fingertips because they can come in handy depending on the particular need you want them to meet.

Scented soy jar candles

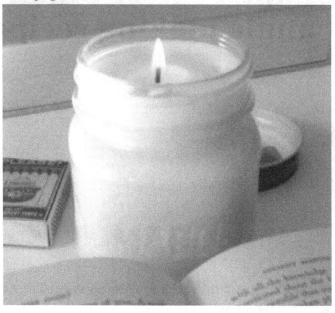

It is important to know that essential oils are used to make this soy candle and not soy candle fragrance oils. You need to use a protective covering like wax paper, plastic tablecloth or newspaper to cover your work surface before you begin. You should also put on cloths that you wouldn't mind if they get messed up. Put aside some paper towel or rags for cleaning up spills. Have all your equipment ready which may include:

Materials

- Wick
- Clean container
- A thermometer
- Stirring rod
- Dye
- Pitcher

Instructions

1. Confirm that the container you want to use is very clean.
2. Take a wick and place it in the center of your jar.
3. You need to heat the jar at this stage. You can use a blow dryer to do this when the wax is ready to be poured in case you have either one or two containers. However, if you have several containers then the easiest way is by warming up to a temperature of 100F in the oven. Don't exceed this temperature in order to prevent them from becoming too hot.
4. It is now time to heat the wax. Take a medium sized pot and pour about 2.5cm equivalent to an inch of water in it. Let it simmer over low heat.
5. Pour the soy wax chips inside a pitcher until it is ¾ full. There are various options you can choose from with regards to the pitcher you can use. You can opt for a large clean reusable can, a heat proof glass pitcher or a metal pitcher.
6. Heat it while stirring until the wax melts completely and gets to about 180F. A thermometer can help you measure this temperature.
7. Add candle dye after the wax has melted. Stir until the dye melts completely and wax achieves a uniform color. It is important to know that a lot of dye is needed for you to achieve a deep color. Therefore, put it in large quantities.
8. Leave the wax for sometime in order to cool down. It should reach a temperature of 140F before adding the essential oil blend you want to use. Stir to enable the oils blend well.
9. Remove your containers from the oven. Group them together to void spills and enable them cool slowly which is important in reducing shrinkage.

10. Pour the wax inside the containers slowly without splashing. This type of slow and even pour helps to prevent the creation of air bubbles.
11. You may need to put aside some wax for recapping in case you want to make a large candle. Recapping simply means re-pouring the candle. After leaving your candle to cool for an hour, you can start poking some holes in the wax to let out the air bubbles. Start with the wax close to the wick. Melt the wax you had reserved and pour some of it in the candle. Be careful not to pour beyond the original fill line. Leave it to cool again.
12. Trim the wick to about 0.5cm equivalent to ¼ inches.

In case you see yourself needing more wax during the melting process then simply add more in to the one already melting and let it all melt together. It is important for the wick to stay in the center to ensure an even burning candle. There are some candle safety precautions you should observe. Don't leave your melting wax unattended. Never heat the wax above a temperature of 275F because it can catch a fire. In case it catches fire then don't pour water on it with the aim of putting out the fire because it will make it spread further. Instead, smother it using a pot lid or baking soda. Never use water-based fragrances or dye when working with wax.

Lavender Race

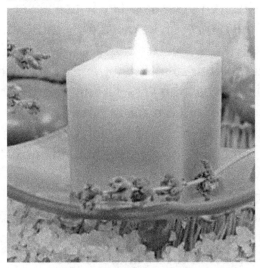

This has a sweet and floral fragrance. This candle can soothe your tired body and calm your anxious mind. It has some lavender flowers and can set the perfect mood for a relaxing evening regardless of the time of the year.

Materials

- Fragrance oil or lavender oil.
- 10 ounces of gel wax. You can use high or medium density Penreco or something similar.
- Liquid oil (this is optional)
- Candlewick and tab
- Some lavender flowers, fresh or dried.
- Toothpicks.
- Small glass containers.
- Heat-proof glass jar.
- Candy thermometer.

Instructions

1. Cut the gel to form small chunks which you can put inside the glass jar. Let it heat over a low flame at a temperature of below 230F until all the pieces have melted.
2. Use the tab to attach an end of the wick to a toothpick lying across the vessel's rim and the remaining end to the bottom of the glass container.
3. Add some drops of liquid color to the melted gel. The liquid color you choose should contrast with that of the lavender flowers.
4. Remove the flame and then add either 20 drops of fragrance oil or 40 drops of lavender essential oil.
5. Gently pour a layer of the gel and allow it to set. This will prevent the formation of bubbles.
6. Sprinkle around 3-4 lavender flowers on top of the setting layer.
7. Add more layers and a few flowers in between the layers until the jar becomes ¾ full.
8. Leave it for around 4-5 hours for the gel to set before trimming the wick to about ¼ inch.

If you want different variations then you can use different colors for the layers. When you add some complementary fragrances like basilicum and pine inside it then you will come up with an exotic combination. Be careful not to add too much fragrance.

Tropical woods

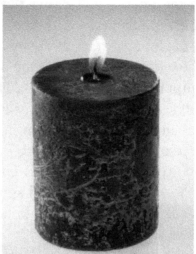

This candle has a woody fragrance that reminds you of green meadows and dark forests stretching out to the horizon. It is made of pure beeswax and gives off a soporific effect as a result of the natural honey notes that exist in the beeswax. You can burn it in your bedroom to enable you have a good night sleep.

Materials

- Double boiler
- 1 lb of beeswax
- Thick candlewick with tab
- Sandalwood fragrance or essential oil
- Metal pudding mold
- Ylang ylang essential oil (this is optional)
- Broomstick
- Silicone spray

Instructions

1. Break the beeswax to form small pieces and put them inside the double boiler. Let the wax completely melt over medium flame.
2. Spray the inner surface of the mold with silicone.
3. Use the tab to fix the wick to the pudding mold's bottom after dipping it inside the wick. The remaining free end should be attached to a broomstick.
4. Get the double boiler away from the flame. Add about 10 drops of the fragrance oil, 10 drops of the ylang ylang oil and 30 drops of the sandalwood oil.
5. Pour the wax inside the mold and let it cool over a cool metal surface. The wax should occupy about ¾ of the vessel.
6. When the sides of the wax have cooled and left some melted wax in the center, it is time to pour out the liquid wax. Do this quickly in order to create a central cavity.
7. Trim the wick to about ¼ inch.
8. The central cavity created will be important in protecting the candle from drafts. This will ensure that it does not go out easily. It is important because lighting beeswax candles is not easy.

Beeswax has an elegant natural color. However, you can add some colors too depending on your preference. Vetiver, cedarwood and rosewood are examples of some of the complementary fragrances you can use. 10 drops of each is enough because they will add up to the required amount of 40 drops.

Zesty Citrus

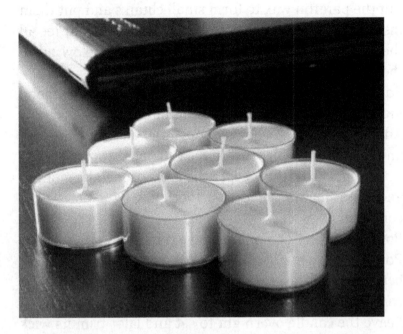

Citrus scents are generally fresh and full of life. You can make your party lively using lots of zesty citrus candles. Paraffin is used to anchor the bright lively colors and the fresh notes.

Materials

- Orange, citronella and lemon fragrance oils.
- 1 lb of paraffin wax.
- 3 small metal jugs
- Liquid colors (yellow, green and orange)
- Candlewick and tabs
- Tall metal or glass containers
- Toothpicks
- Tub of hot water
- Thermometer
- Double boiler

Instructions

1. Cut the paraffin wax to form small chunks and put them inside the double boiler. Apply a low flame and let all the pieces melt ensuring a temperature of below 200F the whole time.
2. Pour about 1/3 of the melted wax inside the three metal jugs and give each of them a different color.
3. Add about 20 drops of every essential oil inside the jugs and mix. Put the jugs inside the tub of hot water.
4. Attach an end of the wick to the glass or metal container and the remaining end to a toothpick lying across the container.
5. Pour one layer of color and leave it to set.
6. Pour other layers of different colors and let the wax set between the layers. Continue doing this until the containers becomes ¾ full.
7. Leave the candle overnight to set and later trim its wick to about ¼ inch.
8. Dip the molds inside hot water and remove them gently to enable the candles unmold.

You can have different variations of this candle if you wish. When you use only two layers, you can come up with two-tone candles. You can get a swirl design when you pour the second layer before the first one is fully set and then use a skewer to mix the layers. In case you want to enhance the fragrance then you can add peppermint or pine oil.

Patchouli Haze

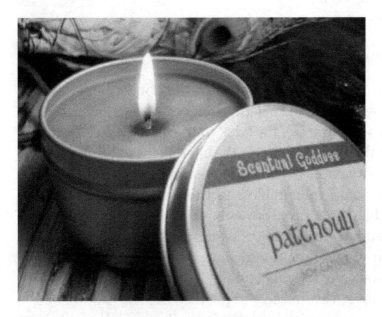

This is an aromatic shrub that is used to make a refreshing essential oil. The candle made from this is great for giving you that cozy feeling especially on either cold or rainy days. When you add some drops of Eucalyptus oil to it then it helps to relieve headaches caused by sinus congestion in addition to decongesting your nostrils. If you are looking for a greener alternative then you can use soy wax.

Materials

- Soy wax chips, 2 lbs
- Eucalyptus oil (this is optional)
- Green color tablets
- Patchouli oil
- Cinnamon oil (this is optional)
- Broomsticks
- Candlewicks with tabs

- Shot glasses
- Double boiler
- Candy thermometer

Instructions

1. Melt the soy wax chips inside the double boiler on low flame. Ensure to keep the temperatures below 220F.
2. Use the tab to fix the wick to the shot glasses' bottoms. Put the broomsticks on the shot glasses and fix the free ends to pieces of these broomsticks.
3. Add some color tablets to the melted wax and stir to enable it dissolve. Soy wax requires lesser amounts of fragrance and color compared to paraffin wax. However, you can add more chips in case you prefer strong colors.
4. Remove the vessel from the flame. Add about 2 tablespoons of the patchouli oil. You can also add about 10 drops of the cinnamon oil to get a sweet note or about 5 drops of the eucalyptus oil if you need a sharper aroma. The cinnamon and the eucalyptus oil are optional.
5. Pour the wax inside the shot glasses gently until they occupy about ¾ of the glasses.
6. Leave it overnight to cool and then trim the wick to about ¼ inch.

If you want a different variation then you can substitute eucalyptus oil with citrus oil.

Peppermint patch

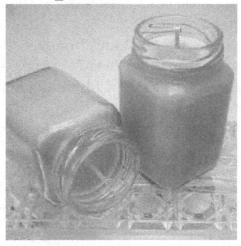

These candles can be used as tea lights and can freshen up your house due to the peppy fragrance they contain. They are very perfect for the holiday festive when you need your home to be full of life.

Materials

- ½ lb of paraffin wax
- Candlewick with tab
- ½ lb of beeswax
- Peppermint fragrance oil or essential oil
- Eggshell halves, metal tart mold and bottle caps
- Toothpicks
- Double boiler

Instructions

1. Break the beeswax to form small pieces which you can add to the paraffin wax granules.
2. Melt this mixture inside a double boiler. Make sure you don't overheat the wax.

3. Use the tab to fix the wick to the mold's bottom after dipping it inside the melted wax. Fix the remaining end to the toothpicks.
4. Take the melted wax away from the flame and add about 40 drops of the oil blend or peppermint oil to it.
5. Pour the wax inside the molds until it almost overflows and then leave it to cool.
6. Use more wax to replenish it in case there were any shrinkage.
7. Let the candles cool and trim the wick to 1/4 inch.

You may add some pine, ginger or palmarosa essential oils to the peppermint oil and blend them to achieve some form of mystery.

Recipes for Moonlight melts massage candles

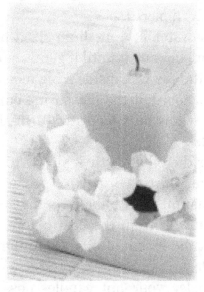

Massage oil candles are amazing due to the fact that they are very good for your skin. In addition to that, they are easy to make and can light up your night in a great way. Massage candles are more than just candles. They are made from body butters and massage oils that melt while the candle burns. They have such a low melting point to the extent that you can pour them on your skin directly without harming it.

Materials

- 1 oz of either Jojoba oil or Sweet Almond oil
- 3 oz of Soy wax
- 4 oz of candle jar or tin
- ½ teaspoons of Vitamin E
- Pre-tabbed candle wick
- 3 drops of the essential oil

Instructions

1. Fix the wick to your candle jar or tin's bottom. (Glue tabs come in handy when doing this. You need to press the glue tabs firmly on the hot wax in order to hold it firmly in place).
2. Pour water in a medium sized pot about an inch high before heating it until it gently simmers.
3. Put the soy wax inside a big measuring cup that is heat-proof too. Put the measuring cup inside the water and give it low heat for it to warm slowly until all the wax melts.
4. Pour the oil and stir it slowly to enable them mix well. Avoid stirring quickly because this will lead to formation of air bubbles in the massage oil candles.
5. Remove it from the heat before adding Vitamin E and then the essential oils. Continue stirring gently all the while.
6. Transfer your hot candle massage oil inside the tin gently while making sure the wick doesn't move from the centre.
7. Leave it for several hours in order for it to cool and harden before trimming the wick to ¼ inch. Your moonlight massage oil candle is ready for use.

When you want to use the massage candle, you need to light it and let the wax gather. You can then pour that melted wax straight on your skin or in your hands before rubbing it on your skin. If you find it too hot then you can give it a minute or two for it to cool down a bit before using it. There are no restrictions with regards to the amount of wax to use. Don't worry if some of the pooled wax hardens in case you don't use it because you can always melt it again to be used next time.

You can customize your massage candles in order to come up with different variations. You can use various carrier oils to speed up or slow down the rate of absorption of the massage oil in to your skin. It can also improve your skin when you do this. You can substitute about an ounce of soy wax with another ounce of cocoa or shea butter. The massage oil candle will come out softer. When you want the massage oil candle to come out harder then you can replace an ounce of soy wax with that of beeswax. Refrain from using dyes with this kind of candle because imagine how you would look like with a green skin or any other color.

Lemon Lavender aromatherapy candle

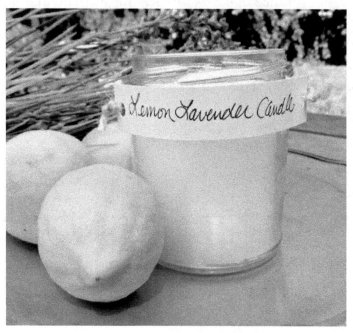

You cannot fail to love the amazing scent of this candle due to the combination of lavender and lemon. It serves to give you a soothing feeling that relaxes your mind and make all your stress melt away.

Ingredients

- 2 ml of lavender and another 2 ml of lemon essential oils
- 6-8 oz of beeswax
- 1 wick
- 4 oz of glass jar
- Pyrex measuring cup.
- 10ml of graduated cylinder. (this is optional)
- Chop sticks
- Small cooking pot

Instructions

1. Measure about 6 oz of the beeswax. You can use 8 oz of if you want the candle to be full to the top.
2. Use jojoba oil to wipe your Pyrex cup.
3. Melt your beeswax inside the Pyrex.
4. Use chop sticks to put the wick inside the jar.
5. Measure the essential oils.
6. Wait for the beeswax to melt before adding the essential oils to it and stirring.
7. Pour the beeswax inside the glass jar slowly and be careful not to interfere with the wick when doing this.
8. Leave it for several hours to solidify.

This combination of lavender and lemon gives out a beautiful scent that reminds you of summer and you can burn them when fall is just setting in order to keep you memories of summer. There are different ways of using this particular candle. You can let it burn in your kitchen as you are taking your morning coffee or tea. You can also burn it when you are having a quiet time reading the bible. You can even burn it when you are just relaxing.

Vanilla soy wax aromatherapy candle

This candle has a pleasant sweet smell that you will love. It can be used by people of all ages from toddlers to adults. It is made using vanilla scent which is known to relax and calm your nervous system. This will therefore relieve you of your anxiety and restlessness. This candle doesn't contain any dyes and can be great for aromatherapy, stress relief, meditation, dance yoga, home décor and general relaxation.

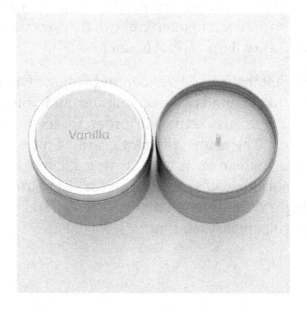

Ingredients

- Skewers
- Vanilla essential oil
- Glass jars. (old candles found in jars can work too)
- Soy wax flakes
- Sticky tape
- Candle fragrance oils
- Candle wicks

Instructions

1. Pour boiling water inside the oil glass candles. Let it cool.
2. Do away with the wax that will be floating on top.
3. Clean up any excess soot or wax using hot water and dishwashing liquid.
4. Dry the glass containers.
5. Cut the sticky tape in to small pieces and fold it to form double sided tape which should be placed in the middle of every jar's bottom.
6. Cut the wicks in such a way that about 4cm of it sticks out of the jar.
7. Press them on the sticky tape with the help of a skewer.
8. Use another skewer to wrap the wick and hold it firmly in the centre.
9. Measure the amount of soy wax flakes you need. It should be double your cup's capacity. For example, 1 cup of candle requires 2 cups of the available soy wax flakes.
10. Put the flakes inside a heat-proof jug before putting it in the microwave for 1 minute.
11. Remove it and stir before putting it back in the microwave for another 1 minute and stirring again.
12. In case some solid flakes are still existing then you can put it back in the microwave for another 20 seconds. Make sure the solid flakes all dissolve.
13. You can now add your fragrance oil, vanilla essential oil and then stir. Pour the wax in the various jars.
14. Confirm that the wicks are still in the centre before leaving it for around 12 hours for it to set
15. Trim the wicks to about 1 inch.

Even though you might see lots of scented candles for sale, they don't compare to the custom made ones that have various fragrances meant to achieve specific moods. Everyone can make them because the procedures are easy and they give you great pleasure while using them. In addition to that, it is quite fun too.

Chapter 4: Fragrances for candle making

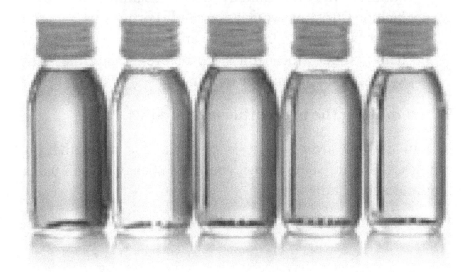

The fragrance you choose for your candle is as important as the process of candle making itself. When learning how to make candles for aromatherapy, it is important to know how to use the various fragrances in order to come up with amazing candles. There are certain components of these fragrances that you should know because they sum up how they are supposed to be used. It is important to know that the fragrances used to make aromatherapy candles are different from the ones used in the various methods of candle making.

Their appeal

Scented candles have been known to have a universal appeal. They do this in various ways:

- ➤ Aromatherapy candles have the ability to bring back old memories. These can range from the memories of a vacation you took to what happened in your childhood.
- ➤ There are some seasonal scents which can be a great addition to your holiday décor. Examples of these include Christmas cookies or candy corn.
- ➤ These candles can boost your energy, calm your nerves, help you get a peaceful sleep or even create the right ambience for a romantic evening.

When making the aromatherapy candles

As fun and rewarding as it is to make the aromatherapy candles, there are some things you need consider when using fragrances for candle making:

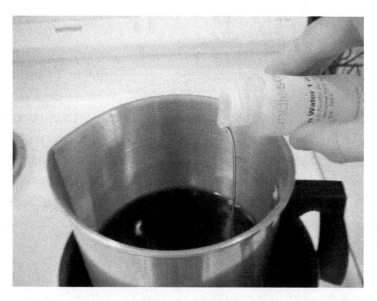

- ➤ It is advisable to buy the best quality fragrance to use for making the candles. Using inferior materials will not give you the quality of candles you desire.

- You need to know how to differentiate essential oils from fragrance oils. Although all of them can be used in aromatherapy candle making, they are not interchangeable. Fragrance oils do not have therapeutic purpose.
- You should know that aromatherapy candles require strong fragrances. You can start by putting some few drops of the fragrances you are using and add more as you proceed according to the required amount. However, make sure you don't over use the fragrance because it will be difficult to try and correct that. Generally you can use less than four ounces of the fragrance for about ten pounds of wax.
- In case you are not able to identify a fragrance that meets your specific needs then you can mix different oils to try and achieve your own blend. It is important to keep records of this in case you want to duplicate those results sometime in the future.

Buying the fragrances used for candle making

You can get the basic supplies for making aromatherapy candles at large craft stores. However, you can also get them online. You can look for those who sell the fragrances you need. Ensure that they are of high quality. You can get some companies that sell quality fragrances at affordable prices.

Other uses of the candle making fragrances

Another great thing about the candle making fragrances is the fact that they can also be used in other crafts. The same supplies are used to make scented linen spray, body lotion, coordinating soaps and homemade potpourri. You can create gift baskets containing complementary items that you can give to your loved ones.

Chapter 5: Instructions to follow during aromatherapy candle making

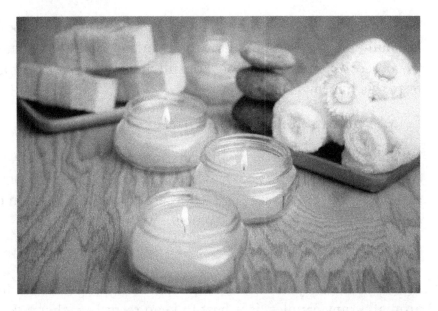

The process of making aromatherapy candles is a unique one. However, it is quite simple if you adhere to the set instructions.

1. Have a clear purpose

It is important to have a clear purpose of what you want to achieve with the aromatherapy candle before you even begin. This is due to the fact that the different candles have different effects. Establish whether you want to relieve some stress, lose weight or any other purpose. This will guide you in to knowing the type of candle to make and the type of essential oil to use.

2. Strong fragrance

You should know that essential oils contain very strong fragrances. It is therefore important to be careful when adding these essential oils to your wax. Start with a few drops and add as you continue with the process.

3. Make Consultations

You need adequate and the right information about aromatherapy candles and how to make them before you start the process. You can therefore consult books and websites that have this information.

4. You can make your formulas

When you have the right information about aromatherapy candles and you practice making them then you will have experience at some point. You will therefore be in a position to even try different blends and come up with your own too.

5. Maintain records

When you find yourself coming up with new formulas for aromatherapy candles, it is best to keep records of them. You never know when you or someone else will need them.

Final thoughts

Aromatherapy dates back to thousands of years when people used candles to create a calm and soothing atmosphere. From that time up to now, there are many people who have tried it and can attest to experiencing positive results.

It has been proven to increase energy levels, treat insomnia and even reduce the pain caused by migraines. This goes to prove that you don't need to have a complicated health problem to require aromatherapy. It can be applied in our day to day lives for something as simple as soothing you to sleep.

There are many stores selling aromatherapy candles and people have been buying them for years. However, you can now make your own by following the guidelines provided in this book. You no longer have an excuse of being dissatisfied with some missing ingredients from your aromatherapy candles because you have the power to choose your own ingredients. In addition to that, it is quite affordable to make your own.

You need to try making and using aromatherapy candles in order to experience its therapeutic benefits first hand.

Yours Sincerely,

Michelle.

Printed in the USA
CPSIA information can be obtained
at www.ICGtesting.com
LVHW020306291223
767719LV00037B/829